2ND EDITION
DIET CHAOS
Lose Weight – Not Your Mind!

DAVID MEINE

Author of *Think: Use Your Mind to Shrink Your Waistline*

Published by David Meine and IdealShape, LLC
921 West 500 North
Lindon, Utah 84042

www.idealshape.com
David's website: www.davidmeine.com
Phone: 1-800-515-0896

ISBN-10: 1495404374 (e)
ISBN-13: 9781495404375 (p)

Dedicated to the IdealShape
community and all those who inspire
others to achieve health and wellness.

CONTENTS

DIET CHAOS

Why Modern Dieting is Doomed to Fail (and How You Can Change It)

Research suggests that up to 95% of dieters regain the weight they lose on a diet.

But you knew that, didn't you? We don't really need statistics to tell us that diets are failing. How many people do you actually know who successfully stuck with a diet long-term?

"The diet business has never been in better shape—unlike many of its customers," a BBC News article reported in 2003. Sadly, not much has changed in a decade.

Today, people around the globe are buying diet programs more desperately than ever—**yet the weight has barely budged.** In fact, we have reached a worldwide obesity crisis.

It's safe to say that the modern method of "going on a diet" isn't working. But why not?

Because diets are doomed to fail from the get-go.

Just like modern furniture and clothing, the modern

diet is built to break. And one thing is for sure: while you may enjoy buying a new couch or outfit every year, jumping from diet to diet isn't fun. In fact, it can be dangerous to your health.

So why aren't diets sustainable?

Because of a concept I call "Diet Chaos."

The components of every standard diet program lead to a state of mental and physical confusion. Stress builds, and this ultimately causes the body to rebel and revert to its original state.

Some people get a few weeks in; others might make it a year on their diet. But inevitably, the mind and body are pushed to a breaking point, and the cycle begins again.

Modern dieting is flawed, but we have the ability to fix it and achieve our health potential.

In this book, I show you how.

But wait—Why hasn't anyone discussed Diet Chaos before?

People want solutions, and diets look like solutions. They promise a quick-fix to all your problems and insist that it's going to happen overnight. The truth--you didn't gain all that weight overnight, and you're not going to lose it overnight. If for some reason you are so successful, the weight loss isn't going to last.

When I began researching the phenomenon I was observing in dieters, I looked to authorities for research on why people were going into a mind-and-body paralysis as they tried to change their eating and exercise behaviors.

I searched for published research from psychologists, dietitians, weight loss experts, medical doctors and college professors, but I found nothing. I was completely surprised (and very disappointed, as I was intending to build on someone else's theories.)

Surely scientists in these fields would have stepped up and exposed Diet Chaos by now! But no. Even our trusted weight loss experts are leading us, whether they realize it or not, down a path of Diet Chaos.

For example, a personal trainer shared with me one of her client's recent experiences. Over the course of one week, she watched Dr. Oz highlight three different weight loss programs on his TV show. Believing that Dr. Oz is the guru on medical advice, this woman was going to try to do **all three diets.** Talk about chaos.

Thankfully, her personal trainer told her that Dr. Oz gets paid to push all those diets, so he wasn't necessarily dispensing objective diet advice.

If you want to achieve weight loss, plain and simple, you'll have to create your own dieting strategy.

Before you consider another diet, read this book.

Successful dieting has two steps:

STEP ONE: Understand mental and physical Diet Chaos.

STEP TWO: Use an approach that eliminates Diet Chaos and creates a clear, consistent path to changing your behavior and body permanently.

I've created such an approach, which I call "The *Think* Method," so you can create your ideal shape for life. I'll explain it to you in this book.

I'll also tell you the magic number of diet changes to make each 28 days, and show you which health habits to focus on for powerful results.

Life is too short to go broke and frazzled in a never-ending diet abyss. Ditch Diet Chaos and start making changes immediately that create permanent nutrition and exercise habits!

CHAPTER 1

What Exactly is Diet Chaos?

When I first introduced the concept of Diet Chaos in my published book *Think: Use Your Mind to Shrink Your Waistline*, I put "and" between the two words: "Diets and Chaos."

I had joined the words to describe what happened with a potential client who came to me for a weight loss consultation. But I hadn't realized just how related the words are.

The woman who contacted me had just started a diet. As part of her diet, she was not only trying to change her eating habits (her goal was to lose 30 pounds in a matter of weeks), but actually trying to change a total of 7 behaviors at the same time.

Unsurprisingly, at least to me, she was frazzled—and she was failing.

In a standard dictionary, "chaos" is defined as follows:

> 1. A condition of great disorder or confusion.
> 2. A disorderly mass; a jumble.
> 3. An abyss; a chasm.

I don't know about you, but all three of those definitions describe my own physical and mental state any time I've been on a diet.

I've always ended up **confused**, with no idea where to start. By trying to focus my effort in so many places, I was rarely effective in any area. (You know what they say about multitasking.) I had a disorderly jumble of "to-dos" on my list, and I wasn't doing any of them well.

I also felt like I was confronted with an **abyss** or **chasm** each time I started a diet. There was a huge gap between what my current body was, and the body shape I wanted to create. It felt like I was diving into the great unknown.

Eventually, the abyss would always spit me back out, and I would end up mentally and physically worse off than before I started the diet.

I jumped on the bandwagon whenever a new, "this one's really it" diet came out—but only to repeat the cycle.

In the end, the result was always a growing sense of discouragement, to accompany my growing waistline.

And then came the 'aha' moment.

Looking at my own experience and that of the dieter who came to me overwhelmed by her 7-part weight loss plan, I realized that chaos was inherent to the dieting process. **Diets ARE chaos.** All require changing too many things at once.

The Laundry List of Diet Rules

Here's what many people put on their to-do lists when they start a diet (and it's by no means conclusive!):

- Reducing calorie intake
- Cutting out certain foods
- Changing beverage choices
- Choosing new exercises
- Seeking emotional support from others
- Cutting back on desserts, candy, and other sweets
- Reading diet books and magazine articles
- Creating some type of tracking system for all the components of the diet
- Diet-proofing the house
- Buying new exercise clothes
- Seeking medical advice from a doctor
- Taking diet supplements
- Increasing caffeine for energy
- Buying a gym membership
- Buying protein drinks
- Preparing more meals at home
- Taking homemade lunches to work or school
- Making meal times more regular
- Checking one's horoscope to see if it's even a good time to start a diet

Changing behaviors is no easy task—it requires a great deal of focus and energy to consciously change an unconscious behavior!

I also came to realize that **the body and brain are resistant to change.** They like homeostasis and will fight to preserve it. Too many changes at once can send off panic alarms, which put the mind and body in a state of chaos.

On top of fatigue, confusion, and irritation in the mind, the body suffers from headaches, withdrawals, cravings, and other side effects.

Have you experienced Diet Chaos? My guess is that if you've gone on any popular diet or weight loss plan, you have.

Take a look at the list on the previous page. Dizzying, right? Now look at it again, and circle each item that you have done at the same time for a past or current diet. Did you circle more than two? More than three? Five? Ten?

If you tried to adopt more than 2 habits at the same time, you likely failed.

Diet Chaos occurs anytime an individual is consciously trying to change more than two behaviors at one time. Just three simultaneous changes can send the brain and body into a tailspin. Yet most of my clients, when they first come to IdealShape, are trying to change five or more things at once while they diet!

The biggest consequence of Diet Chaos is that it **wipes out the tools you need most to succeed** in making changes. Diet Chaos wipes out your mental and physical strength.

Now let's take a closer look at how this actually happens. The following two chapters will define and explain mental and physical diet chaos.

CHAPTER

Defining Mental Diet Chaos

2

Contrary to popular belief, the most stressful thing about dieting isn't giving up your favorite food.

The most stressful thing about dieting is dieting.

What seems, on the surface, like a simple set of rules, in practice becomes complex, unpredictable, and confusing.

The following story will help explain my definition and theory of mental dieting chaos.

In January of 2013, I was skiing at Deer Valley ski resort with one of my best friends, Rogan, whom I've known since college. It was a powder skier's dream: during the previous day and night, it had dumped 14 inches of new snow.

After some awesome runs down open areas, we decided to head over to ski in the trees. To tell the truth, I was scared—in fact, I was completely convinced that I would wreck and seriously injure myself, even though I had skied in the powder among trees for years—but if my friend Rogan wanted to do it, so would I.

On the third run through the trees, I caught my right

ski on a tree and went down. I knew that was going to happen. I was so mad. My body and skis were buried and it took me 20 minutes to get myself out. Though I suffered no serious injuries to my body (fortunately), my psyche was tremendously shaken.

Did you catch what I said in the previous paragraph? That I *knew* I was going to wreck in the trees? My mindset at that moment was that the trees freaked me out and that there were so many of them. My focus was not on the openings between the trees, but the trees themselves.

On top of that, I was worrying about my ski pole plants, shifting the weight on my skis, ducking low tree branches, not being able to see my skis since they were in deep powder, and praying I would not permanently damage my body.

In essence, my mind was in a state of chaos. When I finally came out of the trees, Rogan was waiting for me and let me vent about what happened. Finally, when I had no more to say, he made a very interesting comment. He stated that when he skis he is focused on the **openings between the trees.**

At that moment I realized that my failure stemmed from being focused on the negative (hitting a tree) and not the positive (skiing the openings between the trees). If I put all my focus on doing that one thing—skiing the openings—I could succeed. On the very next ski run, my mental clarity was awesome. The chaotic thinking (anxiety and fear) was gone, and I was filled with a euphoric feeling as I flew through the trees.

What if you could fly through your body-shaping program the same way?

Too often, focusing on all the things we're doing wrong actually prevents us from succeeding. It depletes all our mental energy and focus. But by focusing on only one positive behavioral goal at a time, we can breeze past obstacles and create a mounting sense of confidence and momentum.

Recently, Mary from San Diego decided to start a new diet to lose 20 pounds. In typical fashion, she made the following list of to-do's:

1. Reduce calories by changing the foods she eats
2. Reduce calories by changing beverage choices
3. Buy a weight loss supplement
4. Get a detox wrap
5. Start using her gym membership
6. Hide snacks in her house, just in case she needs a fix
7. Proclaim to family and friends her diet plan
8. Journal her diet journey
9. Stop going to fast food restaurants
10. Stop going to fine dining restaurants
11. Buy new running shoes and start running 3 miles a day, 3 times a week

12. Research articles on the internet that could help with her diet plan
13. Decrease alcohol consumption as a calorie reduction tactic
14. Weigh herself every day to see her progress
15. Pick up current magazines with the latest diet tips

The Fundamental Flaw of Diets

The word 'diet' is used to imply a complete, but short-term, overhaul of a person's eating habits.

When you 'go on a diet' it is presumed that you will eventually 'go off of it' too.

Rather than setting oneself up for lifelong changes and results, dieters get a long set of rules to apply all at once and endure for as long as they can.

Diets are not meant to last. No big surprise: they are rarely endured for very long!

While most of these are great changes to make, tackling the whole list at once has already become overwhelming for Mary. She tells me, "I wake up thinking about all the things I need to change, and go to bed thinking of everything I didn't accomplish." It all overflows into a catch-up list (to add to tomorrow's to-do list.)

Rather than feeling excited to improve her nutrition and fitness a little more each day, Mary feels a growing sense of fear and anxiety.

Fear and anxiety are the first signs of mental chaos. In Mary's case, a very clear picture of mental chaos has begun to appear:

- She goes to bed thinking of everything that was not accomplished. This causes her to lay awake anxiously for a period of time before she is able to fall asleep.

- She wakes up each day with a bigger list of diet to-do's. After several days, the compounding list creates more anxiety.

- She is weighing herself every day. She feels a pang of fear when the needle is not moving down, worried that her efforts won't be successful.

- She is not letting go of the past, but dwelling on prior mistakes and failures. This causes more fear and anxiety.

- Her friends and family ask about how she is doing on her latest diet, and she feels that her progress is being watched and judged.

This is how most diets begin.

Rather than inspiring motivation, they create fear, anxiety, and disappointment in ourselves. **The more we focus on the negative, the more likely we are to crash.**

Now that you can see the picture of mental chaos for Mary, can you relate? If you've been on diets before, does contemplating another diet cause your palms to sweat? Do you feel confused or panicky? Is your heart racing? These conditions can cause adrenaline to be released into the body, which enhances fear and anxiety.

Ultimately, that fear and anxiety open the door for mental chaos. As negativity whirls around in our dieting minds, our confidence and control dwindle.

Goals become less clear, and cravings for comfort food intensify.

Loss of sleep adds to the chaos, leaving us exhausted, with little willpower to resist temptation.

Stress and sleep loss create hormone imbalances, which heighten cravings for fattening food.

This is only the mental component of Diet Chaos. Ready to see what's happening in the body when you go on a diet?

CHAPTER

Defining Physical Diet Chaos

Scientists who study Chaos Theory in physics, biology, and economics state that chaos happens when the present does not necessarily predict the future.

To understand physical dieting chaos, it helps to break down the phrase into two different categories: nutrition and exercise. Let's look at nutrition first.

Say you decide to stop eating desserts, meats, and breads all at once to lose 20 pounds. What do you think will happen after 1 day, 1 week, and 1 month?

With so many variables, it's hard to say for sure. **And therein lies the problem.**

To get an idea of how this plays out in a typical diet regimen, let's create a hypothetical experiment using Mary as our test subject.

Mary, as you may recall, is 20 pounds overweight. Our goal is to determine which behavior will most efficiently help Mary achieve her ideal shape. I want you to picture yourself as the scientist working with me in the following example.

With you and I as scientists with PhDs in nutrition, we decide to design the study with the following questions:

Question 1: What is Mary's expectation of the diet? (How fast does she want to lose the 20 pounds?)

Question 2: What is her motivation to lose 20 pounds?

Question 3: How many days will she have to repeat the same behavior, consistently, to lose 20 pounds?

Question 4: Based on published academic findings, what is a healthy amount of weight to lose per day or week?

Question 5: How many calories are in a pound of fat?

Question 6: How many calories does Mary's body naturally burn per day?

Motivation is a game changer for any successful outcome.

Before we get started, it's important to consider that motivation is usually defined by the reward or benefit acquired for the effort. In order to succeed, the reward must be worth what it takes to achieve it.

*Here are our answers:

Answer 1: Mary's expectation is to lose 20 pounds within the next 2 months.

Answer 2: She is motivated because she wants to fit into her spring and summer clothes.

Answer 3: Mary would have to consistently repeat the same behavior for 60 days to lose 20 pounds within two months.

Answer 4: It is healthy to lose 1–2 pounds per week.

Answer 5: There are 3,500 calories in every pound of fat.

Answer 6: Mary naturally burns 1,685 calories per day.

How did we get these answers? For an extended version of this study, please see the appendix.

Now we're ready to conduct the experiment.

We have our subject, Mary, who normally burns 1,658 calories a day.

To lose **1 pound** a week, she can only consume 1,158 calories per day (3,500 calories in each pound / 7 days each week = 500 calories to lose each day. Also, 1,658 calories burned – 500 calories not eaten to lose weight = 1,158 calories she may consume each day.)

To lose **2 pounds** per week she can only consume 658 calories per day (1,658 calories burned each day - 1000 calories not eaten in order to lose weight.)

Now, as we both sit down with Mary, we share with her all of the data. To set the experiment in motion, we now ask Mary what single behavior she has decided to change that will allow her to reduce her caloric intake by 1,000 calories per day.

We haven't shared with her that at 2 pounds per week, she won't make her goal. But, at this point we just want to determine one behavior that she is going to do consistently, every day, for 60 days.

What a minute, why does Mary look so angry? Quick, let's explain to her how a scientific experiment has to work to have a predictable outcome—we can only have **one variable** or the experiment could end in chaos (or worse, start off in chaos).

Before we get any further, Mary stops us cold by pointing a finger at our faces and says, "What you are asking is ridiculous, I can't achieve my goal by making just one change." I decide at this point to let you respond to her statement. Tentatively, you say:

"Mary, what we are doing is creating an experiment

focusing on changing one negative behavior. We want to see if you can have a predictable outcome. If the experiment is not successful you will know for certain that the negative behavior you worked on was not the reason that you ended up 20 pounds overweight."

You continue: "If you try to change two negative behaviors or more at the same time, the experiment ends in a state of disorder. Diet Chaos means that you don't lose the 20 pounds and you really have no idea why. Further, as scientists we have learned that **changing multiple behaviors at the same time can backfire:** when the body experiences shock or stress, a common response is actually to hold on to fat. You want a predictable outcome, right? You want to step on the scale every day and be down .28 of a pound, right?" Mary responds with a "yes" and we proceed. The next step is for Mary to log everything she eats and drinks for the next week. This will require her to record the weight of each food consumed and the fluid ounces of what she drinks. At this point Mary's eyes are starting to glaze over. She responds by saying this is too much work.

"Okay Mary, that is a valid feeling," we say, "but you want to lose 20 pounds in 2 months, right? Don't you want to lose the weight and keep it off for the rest of your life?"

Hesitantly she agrees but then makes an interesting comment: "I don't really care about the rest of my life, I only care about fitting back into my spring and summer clothes that I have not been able to wear for years."

What's the rush?

Our hypothetical experiment sheds light not only on the physical chaos that ensues in a diet, but also why dieting is so frustrating for most people. Dieters spend years putting on the extra weight and then expect to shed the weight magically in a short period of time. One of my favorite sayings: "Most of life's frustrations are unmet expectations." For all of us, dieting has been truly frustrating because we don't realize our expectations of losing the weight.

Exercise for most dieters can be just as unsettling. Choosing a form of exercise is confusing and is often made more difficult by our busy lifestyles or sedentary lives stuck in front of a television.

Further, when someone goes from sedentarism to a rigorous exercise regimen, the body goes into a state of chaos. Overtraining can result in injury, a weakened immune system, or negation of fitness results. In fact, it's very common for an overzealous new exerciser to catch a cold or other illness that sends them back to square one.

For the past six years I have watched a woman walk past my home almost every day. She does this snow, rain, or shine. Her walk has an elevation change of 700 feet, which is pretty steep. We live on the side of a mountain in Lindon, Utah. In passing I have commented how impressed I am with her consistency to exercise. She just smiles. I have to say that she looks fit and healthy. Somehow she made the positive choice to give her body and brain what they critically need—consistent exercise.

She has also found a way to avoid physical chaos. Her routine is not complicated and she is practicing one behavior that continues to predict that her body will maintain her ideal shape. It's enough to achieve results without causing a burning workout.

I encourage IdealShape clients and customers to find 30 minutes a day, three times a week, to exercise. Doing so is simple and can burn 900 to 1,200 calories a week. Here is the math: if you are trying to lose one pound of fat a week, 900 calories used up by exercise leaves only 2,600 calories to adjust through nutrition. The math is very simple. Diet Chaos makes it overcomplicated. **You can achieve results without sending your body into shock.**

But truth be told, you don't need to worry too much about the physical components of weight loss. Focus on your mind, and the rest will follow effortlessly (continue to chapter 4.)

CHAPTER 4

Focusing More on Your Brain Will Make It Easier to Lose Weight

The real secret to losing weight is understanding your motivation and behaviors at the most basic level: your subconscious mind.

How many times have you thought, "I just need more willpower to lose weight"? Then you find yourself staring at your favorite candy bar, and before you know it, the wrapper is off and you are eating it as fast as you can.

Empty wrapper in hand, you immediately start berating yourself for a lack of willpower.

Self-control is not something that we can simply increase at will.

Neuroscientists tell us that 20% of the calories we expend daily are used by the brain. Every thought and decision we make throughout the day burns up this brain energy. *Willpower is not an unlimited resource.*

Let me give you a perfect example. Bob has a goal to lose 50 pounds, but sleeps poorly and eats very little during the day. After getting home from work at 6:00 pm he faces a crisis. His brain is low on energy due to poor sleep and lack of nutrition. He starves himself all day thinking that doing so will help him to lose weight. But he has an insatiable appetite and before he knows it, he eats and drinks 3,000 calories in a three-hour time period and then goes to bed with a full stomach. He lays in bed awake and angry with himself because of his lack of self-control.

You should quickly realize that Bob depleted most of his willpower by making the decision not to feed his brain during the day.

The brain, like a muscle, can become fatigued when exercised too much. The way our brains cope with the willpower issue is to **automate as much of our decision-making as possible.**

How can this knowledge help you lose weight?

Knowing that many of our behaviors were formed through the automated decision process can help us retrace our steps.

Habits are born based on negative or positive reward. A trigger is created, and once established, becomes an automatic behavior without expending any willpower or mental effort. For this reason, it is critical to understand what behaviors you have created that are causing your body to gain or retain weight.

On the flip-side, you can take advantage of automated decision-making to create positive behaviors. In fact, *getting your subconscious mind to work toward your goals is even more important than conscious willpower.*

Diet Chaos creates lack of willpower for most people by depleting their mental energy. Since our brains are easily overwhelmed, the key to lasting weight loss is to work on one new healthy behavior every 28 days. I always suggest that you start off with the easiest new behavior and use the momentum to work your way up.

With each new, positive behavior, you'll find that you have more brain energy to fuel your willpower. And soon enough, you won't even need willpower.

Willpower is not an issue when you train your brain (subconscious mind where habits are stored) new healthy habits.

In the following chapter I have researched 10 positive behaviors that can truly impact your brain and body in a positive way. I personally used all 10 behaviors to create my ideal shape. Once you have built enough good behaviors, you too will have created your ideal body shape for life.

CHAPTER · · · · · · · · · · · · · · · · 5

The Top 10 Positive Behaviors That Create Permanent Weight Loss

By this point, you understand how to set up your weight loss plan *(by changing one behavior at a time)* to avoid mental and physical Diet Chaos. So it's time to make your smart to-do list!

What behavior should you begin working on first? What is going to help you lose the most possible weight—efficiently and healthily?

That's what I'll tell you in this chapter.

As I've mentioned, this "Diet Chaos" book is a supplemental piece to a book I published in January 2013 called, "Think: Use Your Mind to Shrink Your Waistline." That book was a culmination of my research on the brain and weight loss until now.

When I started studying the brain some 15 years ago, my focus was to find how nutrition, beverages, and exercise affected my ADHD brain. I did not want to use FDA approved drugs that have serious side effects to manage negative symptoms (behavior) from my brain. This research led me to ultimately identify 10 negative behaviors that were affecting my brain, health, and ever-growing waistline.

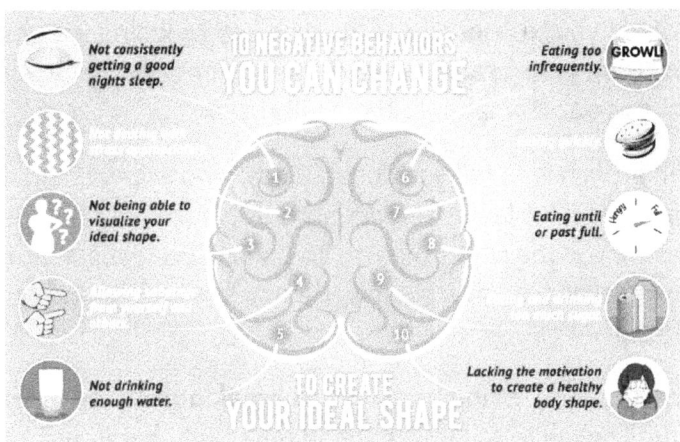

So now you know the negative behaviors. What's the reverse?

Let's look at the 10 positive behaviors you can create to lose weight permanently:

1. Decrease your dependency on sugar
2. Drink more water
3. Get 7 to 8 hours of deep, beneficial sleep
4. Stop weight loss sabotage
5. Learn how to reduce stress
6. Get motivated to exercise
7. Visualize your ideal body shape
8. Eat 5 small meals per day
9. Eat until satisfied and not full
10. Eat slowly to give the brain time to tell you it's full

I want you to understand that **the key to losing weight is using your brainpower.** You should be asking yourself at this point, what does that really mean?

To explain it, I'll tell you about Sandy, who is 52 years old and lives in Atlanta, Georgia. She started working with us at IdealShape when she was 75 pounds overweight. She expressed that she felt powerless to lose weight and get healthy.

Sandy was looking for a way to ***break out of the yoyo dieting cycle,*** but felt she had no way to ***break out of negative behaviors and habits.***

I asked Sandy what she meant when she said she felt powerless. She explained that for the past 30 years she has tried every diet and exercise program with no lasting results. The negative self talk and comforting herself with obscene amounts of sugar was killing her. Borderline diabetes, high blood pressure, and unhealthy cholesterol levels were also taking their toll.

She heard me being interviewed on a radio show, and what caught her attention were the 10 positive behaviors that you could create to lose weight. What stood out the most for her was decreasing dependence on sugar.

Next she was blown away that someone would proclaim that you could focus on creating one positive behavior at a time.

While reading about the Think Method, Sandy learned

that she was drinking **2,500** calories per day from sugary beverages loaded with high fructose corn syrup. That is, *2,500 calories before she had anything to eat.* The Think Method got her to look at everything she ate and drank to figure out how many calories she was consuming from sugar.

And the results are in.

At her body height, age, level of exercise (none), and current weight, Sandy's body only naturally burned 1640 calories. Is it any wonder that she gained weight and felt powerless to change?

The Think Method gave her the mental strength to reach her goal of losing 75 pounds.

The key for her has been mastering one behavior at a time and then building a new positive behavior onto those that she has mastered. She has already created three new positive behaviors: she has decreased her dependence on sugar, gone from consistently poor sleep to 7-8 hours a night, and drinks water as her only beverage of choice.

In the first 4 months, Sandy has lost 35 pounds. What is amazing is that she now believes she is no longer powerless and her self-image has skyrocketed. Before long she will create her ideal body shape for the rest of her life.

It takes brainpower to change negative behaviors.

A list of diet rules, on its own, will never be enough to help us reach our goals.

Over our lifetime we unknowingly or knowingly train (or have trained) our brains to accept a negative behavior as status quo. I listen to clients give 5 to 15 minutes of excuses about why they cannot change their negative behavior. What they are really saying is that they are scared of change or don't want to go through the pain of change, even though the negative behavior is wreaking havoc on their lives.

The brain is so powerful and has amazing resources. Approximately **80% of the brain is subconscious** and is connected to the nervous system that goes throughout the whole body. You don't consciously have to think about breathing, walking, writing, or pressing keys on a keyboard. You have consciously trained your brain how to do all those things, and now they have turned into habits residing at the subconscious level.

You absolutely have the power to retrain your brain. It's your choice to accept or reject a bad behavior. The subconscious mind has been trained to immediately react to a situation that has been experienced and accepted before.

Over time we forget that we have accepted and trained

our brains for negative behaviors, such as not sleeping 7-8 hours a night. When I challenge a client or simply ask about their sleeping pattern, they respond by saying "that is just the way it is." I respond back by explaining that they made a conscious choice to accept not sleeping as a normal behavior. But don't worry!

What you train, you can un-train in the human mind—this ability is innate in us!

The key to training the brain—and avoiding Diet Chaos—is focusing on one new positive behavior at a time.

Let me conclude by going back to the story I shared about my skiing experience. If Rogan had told me three or five things that I would need to do in order to successfully ski in powder through the trees, my fear and anxiety would have increased.

Gratefully on that next ski run I only had to focus on one behavior and that was pointing my skis through the openings between the trees. By changing that one negative behavior of focusing on the trees to the new behavior of focusing on the open spaces, I experienced a paradigm shift.

I have skied 50 to 60 times through the trees for the remainder of the 2013 ski season. Guess what? I haven't hit one tree.

In just 28 days, you can have a habit for life.

Focusing a small amount of time each day—for four weeks—is all it takes to create a positive behavior or habit that sticks.

The surprise bonus: you'll actually reach your goals FASTER by taking it one habit/behavior at a time. You'll avoid Diet Chaos!

So ditch your "diet," and go to FREE Audio Training.

Now you can eliminate Diet Chaos and be a part of the healthy living revolution!

Join David's latest conversation about weight loss and nutrition!

 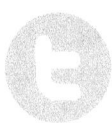 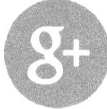  

APPENDIX

Chapter 3 Extended Study:
Continued from page 18

Starting with question 1: Let's ask Mary how long she thinks it will take to lose 20 pounds. Her response is energetic and she states that it will only take two months.

Then we ask her question 2: Ok Mary, what is your motivation for losing the 20 pounds? Her response is that she wants to fit back into her spring and summer clothes. Somehow in her mind she knows that those clothes fit 20 less pounds ago.

Formulas for Question 3:

1. Mary's two month goal means 0 consecutive days.

2. Next divide 20 pounds by 60 days. This equals .33 lbs. per day.

3. Since the government standard for a healthy weight loss range is 1–2 pounds per week, we can compare Mary's goal against this standard. We have 2 formulas to create for healthy weight loss at 1 to 2 lbs. per week:

    a. We take 1 pound per week, divide it by 7 days, and we get .14 lbs.

b. We take 2 pounds per week, divide it by 7 days, and we get .28 lbs.

Here we spot our first red flag: Not even the ambitious end of healthy weight loss will meet Mary's goal of losing 20 pounds in 2 months or .33 pounds every day.

But we'll worry about that discrepancy later. Next we need to find out what Mary will have to do in order to drop those pounds.

Formulas for Question 4:

How many calories are in a pound of fat? Mayo Clinic website states that there are 3,500 calories in a pound of fat. Based on that information, we can create the following formulas:

1. To lose 1 pound per week: Multiply 3,500 calories by 1 and get 3,500 calories. Divide 3,500 calories by 7 days and get 500 calories. Mary would need to reduce her intake by 500 calories per day.

2. To lose 2 pounds per week: Multiply 3,500 calories by 2 and get 7,000 calories. Divide 7000 by 7 days and get 1,000 calories. Mary would need to reduce her intake by 1000 calories per day.

Formulas for Question 5:

How many calories does Mary's body naturally burn per day? To answer this, we have to ask Mary a subset of questions.

5a. How tall is Mary?

5b. Does Mary exercise? If so, how often: We have to ask Mary a subset of questions on this one.

> **5b-1.** Does she currently exercise 1 day per week for 30 minutes?

> **5b-2**. Does she currently exercise 2 days per week for 30 minutes each time?

5c. How much does Mary weigh right now? (You get to ask her that one!)

5d. How old is Mary? (You definitely get to ask her that question!)

Mary gives us the following answers: she is 5'6", rarely exercises (but goes with 1 day per week), currently weighs 155 pounds, and is 42 years old. We take all of that data and put it into the U.S. government calorie calculator, and out pops 1,658—the number of calories she naturally burns per day.

As you recall from Chapter 3, Mary's expectation of losing 20 pounds in two months was not realistic. It would require burning 1,250 calories per day *more* than she consumed. That means if she consumed 1,000 calories, she would have to burn 2,250!

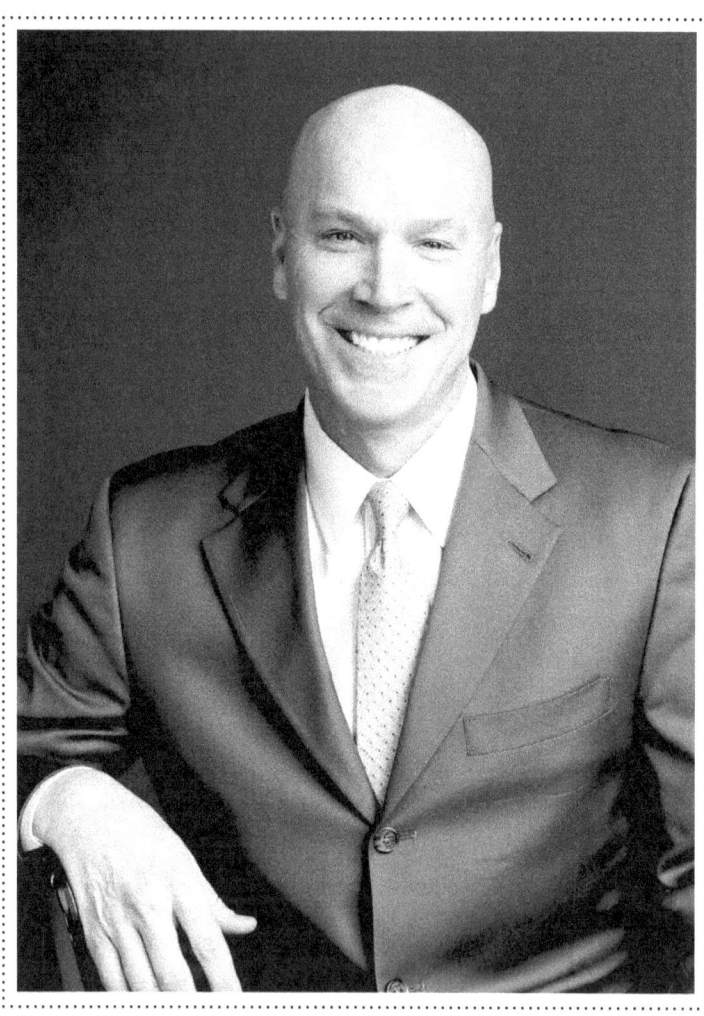

ABOUT THE AUTHOR

David Meine has motivated thousands of people over 30-plus years to create positive thinking behaviors and has now turned his gift toward helping people understand that "permanent weight loss begins and ends in the mind."

He teaches that you are not powerless against the "obesity epidemic" or products of your fast-paced lifestyles. Now he is providing the tools you need to reverse deep-rooted negative thoughts and habits holding you back from attaining lifelong health and wellbeing.

David is the author of *Think: Use Your Mind to Shrink Your Waistline*. He also co-authored the book *IdealShape for Life*, a step-by-step guide to making health and fitness changes that will last a lifetime. He is the creator of an audio motivational weight loss training program for effective weight loss. Try Motivational Weight Loss Training for free.

In 2003 David and his wife Carla co-founded IdealShape, a company that creates weight loss tools including meal replacement shakes, meal replacement bars, nutritional weight loss supplementation, free webinars, books, and exercise programs. David and Carla have 7 children and 10 grandchildren and live in Lindon, Utah.

Learn more from David's website or full biography:
www.davidmeine.com or about.me/david_meine

Think: Use Your Mind to Shrink Your Waistline

In *Think: Use Your Mind to Shrink Your Waistline*, I go deeper into the science behind the brain and help you understand how your mind can be your most powerful ally in achieving your health goals.

In *Think*, I focus on the ten behaviors in detail and explain why they prevent you from losing weight and keeping it off.

Think packs a toolbox filled with techniques to make your weight loss goals become reality. I tell stories and share life examples. I'll help you understand how negative habits are formed and how you can change them at the deepest, most permanent levels of your subconscious mind through motivational weight loss training—one of the most popular new approaches to weight loss.

I show you how to get your mind "in the game" to achieve health, confidence, and the ideal shape you desire.

Get *Think: Use Your Mind to Shrink Your Waistline*.

10 Negative Behaviors You Can
Change to Create Your Ideal Shape

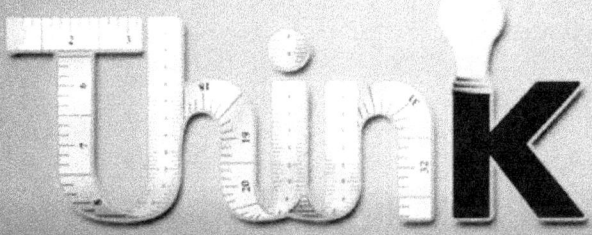

Use Your Mind to Shrink Your Waistline

DAVID MEINE